MEDITERRANEAN COOKBOOK FOR BEGINNERS

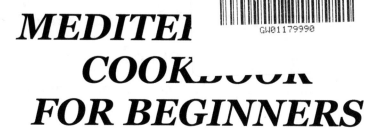

THE COMPLETE MEDITERRANEAN

COOKBOOK FOR BEGINNERS

Helen Harper

© Copyright 2021 - Helen Harper - All rights reserved.

The content contained within this book may not be reproduced, duplicated or transmitted without direct written permission from the author or the publisher.

Under no circumstances will any blame or legal responsibility be held against the publisher, or author, for any damages, reparation, or monetary loss due to the information contained within this book. Either directly or indirectly.

Legal Notice:

This book is copyright protected. This book is only for personal use. You cannot amend, distribute, sell, use, quote or paraphrase any part, or the content within this book, without the consent of the author or publisher.

Disclaimer Notice:

Please note the information contained within this document is for educational and entertainment purposes only. All effort has been executed to present accurate, up to date, and reliable, complete information. No warranties of any kind are declared or implied. Readers acknowledge that the author is not engaging in the rendering of legal, financial, medical or professional advice. The content within this book has been derived from various sources. Please consult a licensed professional before attempting any techniques outlined in this book.

By reading this document, the reader agrees that under no circumstances is the author responsible for any losses, direct or indirect, which are incurred as a result of the use of information contained within this document, including, but not limited to, — errors, omissions, or inaccuracies.

TABLE OF CONTENT

INTRODUCTION 7

RECIPES.. 9

OVERNIGHT BERRY CHIA OATS 10

CINNAMON ROLL OATS 12

CHOCOLATE BANANA SMOOTHIE 14

QUINOA BOWL..15

MEDITERRANEAN BREAKFAST SALAD 17

AVOCADO MILK SHAKE 19

TOMATO AND DILL FRITTATA 20

PROTEIN-PACKED BLENDER PANCAKES........................... 22

PEARL COUSCOUS SALAD.. 24

DELICIOUS FRITTATA WITH BRIE AND BACON 27

QUINOA CHICKEN SALAD.. 29

TASTY TUNA SALAD...31

SHRIMPS COBB SALAD... 33

SWEETEST SWEET POTATO SALAD 35

BRUSSEL PECORINO PINE SALAD...................................... 37

A REFRESHING DETOX SALAD 39

CRAB MELT WITH AVOCADO AND EGG 41

ITALIAN MEATBALL SOUP 43

DILL FARRO 45

TUSCAN CABBAGE SOUP 47

CREAMY CHICKEN-SPINACH SKILLET 49

BEEF AND BULGUR MEATBALLS 51

SIMPLE AND QUICK STEAK.. 53

MEDITERRANEAN GRILLED PORK CHOPS 55

FOUR-CHEESE ZUCCHINI NOODLE WITH BASIL PESTO 57

PORK AND GREENS SALAD 59

MUSTARD CHOPS WITH APRICOT-BASIL RELISH 61

SLOW COOKED MEDITERRANEAN PORK 63

HEARTY BEEF RAGU 65

TURKEY MEATBALLS 67

GARLIC CAPER BEEF ROAST... 69

KALE SPROUTS AND LAMB 71

BEANLESS BEEF CHILI 73

CLASSIC CHICKEN COOKING WITH TOMATOES AND TAPENADE 75

BEEF SHAWARMA 77

MEDITERRANEAN LAMB CHOPS 79

LAMB AND BEET MEATBALLS 81

BEEF AND POTATOES 83

BEEF AND CHILI MIX 85

SALMON AND EGGS 86

GRILLED CALAMARI WITH LEMON JUICE 88

TASTY TUNA WITH ROAST POTATOES 90

SEAFOOD RISOTTO 92

COCONUT SHRIMP 94

ALMOND-CRUSTED SWORDFISH 96

CREAMY AIR FRYER SALMON 99

PEANUT BUTTER AND CHOCOLATE BALLS 101

PEACH CAKE 103

MASCARPONE AND FIG CROSTINI 105

CHOCOLATE MINI CHEESECAKES 107

Introduction

The Mediterranean diet is a nutritional model inspired by the traditional eating styles of the countries bordering the Mediterranean Sea. Scientists from all over the world have been studying it since the 50s of the last century and still today it remains among the diets that, associated with correct lifestyles, have a positive influence on our health.

The Mediterranean diet is a lifestyle, more than just a list of foods. At the base of the food pyramid, there are many vegetables, some fruits, and cereals (preferably whole grains). Going up, we find milk and low-fat derivatives (such as yogurt) contemplated in 2-3 portions of 125ml. Extra virgin olive oil to be consumed raw without exaggerating (3-4 tablespoons per day), together with garlic, onion, spices, and aromatic herbs, instead of salt, are the best condiments for our Mediterranean style dishes. Other good fats in addition to those of oil are provided by nuts and olives, in one or two portions of 30g.

Towards the top of the food pyramid, there are foods to be consumed not every day, but weekly: they are the ones which mainly provide proteins, among which we should favor fish and legumes with at least two portions per week each, poultry 2-3 portions, eggs from 1 to 4 per week, cheeses not more than a couple of 100g portions, 50g if they are aged.

At the top of the pyramid, there are also foods to be consumed in moderation: two portions or less per week for red meat (100g), while processed meats (cold cuts, salami, etc..) should be consumed even more sparingly (one portion per week of 50g or less). Finally, sweets should be consumed as little as possible.

RECIPES

Overnight Berry Chia Oats

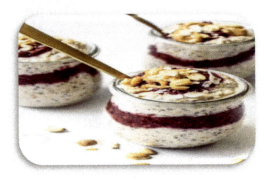

Prep Time: 15 mins **Cook Time:** 5 mins **Total Time:** 20 mins

MAKES 1 SERVING

INGREDIENTS

- ✓ 1/2 cup Quaker Oats rolled oats
- ✓ 1/4 cup chia seeds
- ✓ 1 cup milk or water
- ✓ pinch of salt and cinnamon
- ✓ maple syrup, or a different sweetener, to taste
- ✓ 1 cup frozen berries of choice or smoothie leftovers

Toppings:

- ✓ Yogurt Berries

INSTRUCTIONS

1. In a jar with a lid, add the oats, seeds, milk, salt, and

cinnamon, refrigerate overnight. On serving day, puree the berries in a blender.
2. Stir the oats, add in the berry puree and top with yogurt and more berries, nuts, honey, or garnish of your choice. Enjoy!

Cinnamon Roll Oats

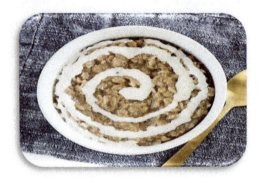

Prep Time: 7 mins **Cook Time:** 10 mins **Total Time:** 17 mins

MAKES 4 SERVINGS

INGREDIENTS

- ½ cup rolled oats 1 cup milk
- 1 teaspoon vanilla extract
- 1 teaspoon ground cinnamon
- 2 teaspoon honey
- 2 tablespoons Plain yogurt
- 1 teaspoon butter

INSTRUCTIONS

1. Pour milk into the saucepan, then bring it to a boil. Add rolled oats and stir well.
2. Close the lid and simmer the oats for 5 minutes over medium heat. The cooked oats will absorb all milk.

3. Then, add butter and stir the oats well.
4. In the separated bowl, whisk together Plain yogurt with honey, cinnamon, vanilla extract.
5. Transfer the cooked oats to the serving bowls.
6. Top the oats with the yogurt mixture in the shape of the wheel.

Chocolate Banana Smoothie

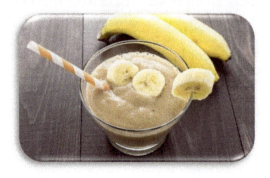

Prep Time: 5 mins **Cook Time:** 0 mins **Total Time:** 5 mins

MAKES 2 SERVINGS

INGREDIENTS

- ✓ 2 bananas, peeled
- ✓ 1 cup unsweetened almond milk, or skim milk
- ✓ 1 cup crushed ice
- ✓ 3 tablespoons unsweetened cocoa powder
- ✓ 3 tablespoons honey

INSTRUCTIONS

1. In a blender, combine the bananas, almond milk, ice, cocoa powder, and honey. Blend until smooth.

Quinoa Bowl

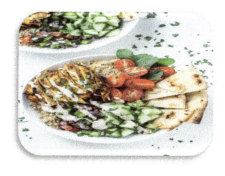

Prep Time: 10 mins **Cook Time:** 20 mins **Total Time:** 30 mins

MAKES 4 SERVINGS

INGREDIENTS

- ✓ 1 sweet potato, peeled, chopped
- ✓ 1 tablespoon olive oil
- ✓ ½ teaspoon chili flakes
- ✓ ½ teaspoon salt
- ✓ 1 cup quinoa
- ✓ 2 cups of water
- ✓ 1 teaspoon butter
- ✓ 1 tablespoon fresh cilantro, chopped

INSTRUCTIONS

1. Line the baking tray with parchment.
2. Arrange the chopped sweet potato in the tray and

sprinkle it with chili flakes, salt, and olive oil.
3. Bake the sweet potato for 20 minutes at 355F. Meanwhile, pour water into the saucepan.
4. Add quinoa and cook it over medium heat for 7 minutes or until quinoa will absorb all liquid.
5. Add butter in the cooked quinoa and stir well.
6. Transfer it to the bowls, add the baked sweet potato, and chopped cilantro.

Mediterranean Breakfast Salad

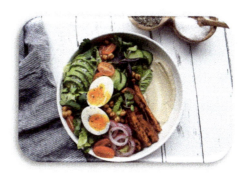

Prep Time: 15 mins **Cook Time:** 10 mins **Total Time:** 25 mins

MAKES 2 SERVINGS

INGREDIENTS

- ✓ 4 eggs (optional)
- ✓ 10 cups arugula
- ✓ 1/2 seedless cucumber, chopped
- ✓ 1 cup cooked quinoa, cooled
- ✓ 1 large avocado
- ✓ 1 cup natural almonds, chopped
- ✓ 1/2 cup mixed herbs, chopped
- ✓ 2 cups halved cherry tomatoes and/or heirloom tomatoes cut into wedges
- ✓ Extra virgin olive oil
- ✓ 1 lemon
- ✓ Sea salt, to taste
- ✓ Freshly ground black pepper, to taste

INSTRUCTIONS

1. Cook the eggs by soft-boiling them - Bring a pot of water to a boil, then reduce heat to a simmer. Gently lower all the eggs into the water and allow them to simmer for 6 minutes.
2. Remove the eggs from water and run cold water on top to stop the cooking, the process set aside, and peel when ready to use.
3. In a large bowl, combine the arugula, tomatoes, cucumber, and quinoa. Divide the salad among 2 containers, store in the fridge for 2 days.

Avocado Milk Shake

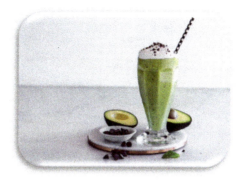

Prep Time: 10 mins **Cook Time:** 0 mins **Total Time:** 10 mins

MAKES 3 SERVINGS

INGREDIENTS

- ✓ 1 avocado, peeled, pitted
- ✓ 2 tablespoons of liquid honey
- ✓ ½ teaspoon vanilla extract
- ✓ ½ cup heavy cream
- ✓ 1 cup milk
- ✓ 1/3 cup ice cubes

INSTRUCTIONS

1. Chop the avocado and put in the food processor.
2. Add liquid honey, milk, vanilla extract, heavy cream, and ice cubes. Blend the mixture until it smooth.
3. Pour the cooked milkshake in the serving glasses.

Tomato and Dill Frittata

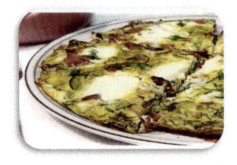

Prep Time: 5 mins **Cook Time:** 10 mins **Total Time:** 15 mins

MAKES 4 SERVINGS

INGREDIENTS

- ✓ 2 tablespoons olive oil
- ✓ 1 medium onion, chopped
- ✓ 1 teaspoon garlic, minced
- ✓ 2 medium tomatoes, chopped
- ✓ 6 large eggs
- ✓ ½ cup half and half
- ✓ ½ cup feta cheese, crumbled
- ✓ ¼ cup dill weed Salt as needed
- ✓ Ground black pepper as needed

INSTRUCTIONS

1. Pre-heat your oven to a temperature of 400 degrees Fahrenheit. Take a large-sized ovenproof pan and heat

your olive oil over medium-high heat. Toss in the onion, garlic, tomatoes and stir fry them for 4 minutes.
2. While they are being cooked, take a bowl and beat together your eggs, half and half cream, and season the mix with some pepper and salt.
3. Pour the mixture into the pan with your vegetables and top it with crumbled feta cheese and dill weed. Cover it with the lid and let it cook for 3 minutes.
4. Place the pan inside your oven and let it bake for 10 minutes. Serve hot.

Protein-Packed Blender Pancakes

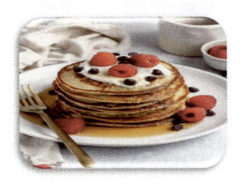

Prep Time: 5 mins **Cook Time:** 10 mins **Total Time:** 15 mins

MAKES 1 SERVING

INGREDIENTS

- ✓ 2 organic eggs
- ✓ 1 scoop protein powder
- ✓ Salt to taste
- ✓ ¼ tsp cinnamon
- ✓ 2oz cream cheese, softened
- ✓ 1 tsp unsalted butter

INSTRUCTIONS

1. Crack the eggs in a blender, add remaining ingredients except for butter, and pulse for 2 minutes until well combined and blended.
2. Take a skillet pan, place it over medium heat, add butter

and when it melts, pour in prepared batter, spread it evenly, and cook for 4 to 5 minutes per side until cooked through and golden brown.

Pearl Couscous Salad

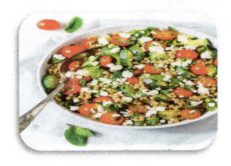

Prep Time: 15 mins **Cook Time:** 0 mins **Total Time:** 15 mins

MAKES 6 SERVINGS

INGREDIENTS

For Lemon Dill Vinaigrette:

- Juice of 1 large-sized lemon
- 1/3 cup of extra virgin olive oil
- 1 teaspoon of dill weed
- 1 teaspoon of garlic powder
- Salt as needed
- Pepper

For Israeli Couscous:

- 2 cups of Pearl Couscous
- Extra virgin olive oil
- 2 cups of halved grape tomatoes

- ✓ Water as needed
- ✓ 1/3 cup of finely chopped red onions
- ✓ ½ of a finely chopped English cucumber
- ✓ 15 ounces of chickpeas
- ✓ 14 ounce can of artichoke hearts (roughly chopped up)
- ✓ ½ cup of pitted Kalamata olives
- ✓ 15-20 pieces of fresh basil leaves, roughly torn and chopped up
- ✓ 3 ounces of fresh baby mozzarella

INSTRUCTIONS

1. Prepare the vinaigrette by taking a bowl and add the ingredients listed under the vinaigrette. Mix them well and keep them aside. Take a medium-sized heavy pot and place it over medium heat.
2. Add 2 tablespoons of olive oil and allow it to heat up. Add couscous and keep cooking until golden brown. Add 3 cups of boiling water and cook the couscous according to the package instructions.
3. Once done, drain in a colander and keep aside. Take another large-sized mixing bowl and add the remaining ingredients except for the cheese and basil.
4. Add the cooked couscous and basil to the mix and mix everything well. Give the vinaigrette a nice stir, then whisk it into the couscous salad. Mix well.

5. Adjust the seasoning as required. Add mozzarella cheese. Garnish with some basil. Enjoy!

Delicious Frittata with Brie and Bacon

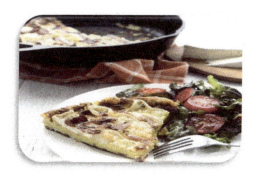

Prep Time: 10 mins **Cook Time:** 20 mins **Total Time:** 30 mins

MAKES 2 SERVINGS

INGREDIENTS

- ✓ 4 slices of bacon
- ✓ 4 organic eggs, beaten
- ✓ ½ cup heavy cream
- ✓ Salt and freshly cracked black pepper, to taste
- ✓ 4 oz brie, diced
- ✓ 1 ½ cup of water
- ✓ 1 tbsp olive oil

INSTRUCTIONS

1. Switch on the instant pot, insert its inner pot, press the 'sauté' button, and when hot, add bacon slices and cook

for 5 to 7 minutes until crispy.
2. Then transfer bacon to a plate lined with paper towels to drain grease and set aside until required.
3. Crack eggs in a bowl, add cream, season with salt and black pepper and whisk until combined.
4. Chop the cooked bacon, add to the eggs along with brie and stir until mixed. Take a baking dish, grease it with oil, pour in the egg mixture, and spread evenly.
5. Carefully pour water into the instant pot, insert a trivet stand, place baking dish on it, shut with lid, then press the 'manual' button and cook the frittata for 20 minutes at a high-pressure setting.
6. When the timer beeps, press the 'cancel' button, allow pressure to release naturally until the pressure valve drops, then open the lid and take out the baking dish.
7. Wipe clean moisture on top of the frittata with a paper towel and let it cool completely.
8. For meal prep, cut frittata into six slices, then place each slice in a plastic bag or airtight container and store in the refrigerator for up to three days or store in the freezer until ready to eat.

Quinoa Chicken Salad

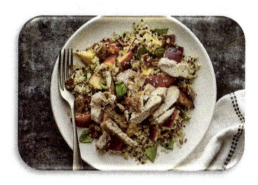

Prep Time: 15 mins **Cook Time:** 20 mins **Total Time:** 35 mins

MAKES 8 SERVINGS

INGREDIENTS

- ✓ 2 cups of water
- ✓ 2 cubes of chicken bouillon
- ✓ 1 smashed garlic clove
- ✓ 1 cup of uncooked quinoa
- ✓ 2 large-sized chicken breasts cut up into bite-sized portions and cooked
- ✓ 1 large-sized diced red onion
- ✓ 1 large-sized green bell pepper
- ✓ ½ cup of Kalamata olives
- ✓ ½ cup of crumbled feta cheese
- ✓ ¼ cup of chopped up parsley
- ✓ ¼ cup of chopped up fresh chives

- ✓ ½ teaspoon of salt
- ✓ 1 tablespoon of balsamic vinegar
- ✓ ¼ cup of olive oil

INSTRUCTIONS

1. Take a saucepan and bring your water, garlic, and bouillon cubes to a boil. Stir in quinoa and reduce the heat to medium-low.
2. Simmer for about 15-20 minutes until the quinoa has absorbed all the water and is tender. Discard your garlic cloves and scrape the quinoa into a large-sized bowl.
3. Gently stir in the cooked chicken breast, bell pepper, onion, feta cheese, chives, salt, and parsley into your quinoa.
4. Drizzle some lemon juice, olive oil, and balsamic vinegar. Stir everything until mixed well. Serve warm and enjoy!

Tasty Tuna Salad

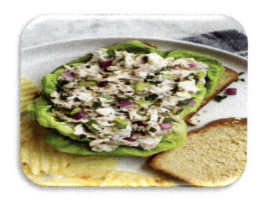

Prep Time: 15 mins **Cook Time:** 0 mins **Total Time:** 15 mins

MAKES 4 SERVINGS

INGREDIENTS

Salsa Verde Chicken

- ✓ Green olives - 1 4 cups, sliced
- ✓ Tuna in water - 1 can, drained
- ✓ Pine nuts - 2 tbsp.
- ✓ Artichoke hearts – 1 jar, drained and chopped
- ✓ Extra virgin olive oil - 2 tbsp.
- ✓ Lemon – 1, juiced
- ✓ Arugula - 2 leaves
- ✓ Dijon mustard - 1 tbsp.
- ✓ Salt and pepper - to taste

INSTRUCTIONS

1. Mix mustard, oil, and lemon juice in a bowl to make a dressing. Combine the artichoke hearts, tuna, green olives, arugula, and pine nuts in a salad bowl.
2. In a separate salad bowl, mix tuna, arugula, pine nuts, artichoke hearts, and tuna.
3. Pour dressing mix onto the salad and serve fresh.

Shrimps Cobb Salad

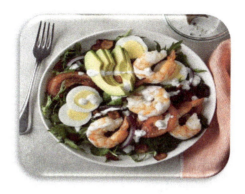

Prep Time: 25 mins **Cook Time:** 10 mins **Total Time:** 35 mins

MAKES 2 SERVINGS

INGREDIENTS

- ✓ 4 slices center-cut bacon
- ✓ 1 lb. large shrimp, peeled and deveined
- ✓ 1/2 teaspoon ground paprika
- ✓ 1/4 teaspoon ground black pepper
- ✓ 1/4 teaspoon salt, divided
- ✓ 2 1/2 tablespoons. Fresh lemon juice
- ✓ 1 1/2 tablespoons. Extra-virgin olive oil
- ✓ 1/2 teaspoon whole grain Dijon mustard
- ✓ 1 (10 oz.) package romaine lettuce hearts, chopped
- ✓ 2 cups cherry tomatoes, quartered
- ✓ 1 ripe avocado, cut into wedges
- ✓ 1 cup shredded carrots

INSTRUCTIONS

1. In a large skillet over medium heat, cook the bacon for 4 minutes on each side till crispy. Take away from the skillet and place on paper towels; let cool for 5 minutes. Break the bacon into bits.
2. Pour out most of the bacon fat, leaving behind only 1 tablespoon. in the skillet. Then, bring the skillet back to medium-high heat.
3. Add black pepper and paprika to the shrimp for seasoning. Cook the shrimp for around 2 minutes on each side until it is opaque. Sprinkle with 1/8 teaspoon of salt for seasoning.
4. Combine the remaining 1/8 teaspoon of salt, mustard, olive oil, and lemon juice in a small bowl. Stir in the romaine hearts.
5. On each serving plate, place 1 and 1/2 cups of romaine lettuce. Add on top the same amounts of avocado, carrots, tomatoes, shrimp, and bacon.

Sweetest Sweet Potato Salad

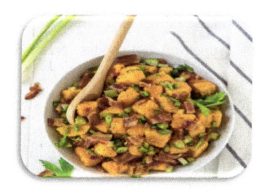

Prep Time: 10 mins **Cook Time:** 20 mins **Total Time:** 30 mins

MAKES 4 SERVINGS

INGREDIENTS

- ✓ Honey - 2 tbsp.
- ✓ Sumac spice - 1 tsp.
- ✓ Sweet potato - 2, finely sliced
- ✓ Extra virgin olive oil - 3 tbsp.
- ✓ Dried mint - 1 tsp.
- ✓ Balsamic vinegar – 1 tbsp.
- ✓ Salt and pepper - to taste
- ✓ Pomegranate - 1, seeded
- ✓ Mixed greens - 3 cups

INSTRUCTIONS

1. Place sweet potato slices on a plate and add sumac, mint, salt, and pepper on both sides. Next, drizzle oil and honey over both sides.
2. Add oil to a grill pan and heat. Grill sweet potatoes on medium heat until brown on both sides.
3. Put sweet potatoes in a salad bowl and top with pomegranate and mixed greens.
4. Stir and eat right away.

Brussel Pecorino Pine Salad

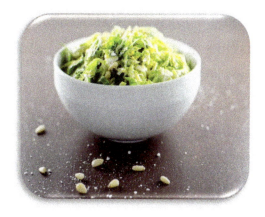

Prep Time: 15 mins **Cook Time:** 0 mins **Total Time:** 15 mins

MAKES 4-6 SERVINGS

INGREDIENTS

- ¼ cup extra-virgin olive oil
- ¼ cup pine nuts, toasted
- 1 garlic clove, minced
- 1 pound Brussels sprouts, trimmed, halved, and sliced thin
- 1 small shallot, minced
- 1 tablespoon Dijon mustard
- 2 ounces Pecorino Romano cheese, shredded (2/3 cup)
- 2 tablespoons lemon juice
- Salt and pepper

INSTRUCTIONS

1. Beat lemon juice, mustard, shallot, garlic, and ½ teaspoon salt together in a big container. Whisking continuously, slowly drizzle in oil.
2. Put in Brussels sprouts, toss to coat, and allow to sit for a minimum of half an hour or a maximum of 2 hours. Mix in Pecorino and pine nuts. Sprinkle with salt and pepper. Serve.

A Refreshing Detox Salad

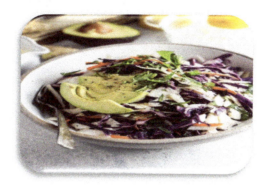

Prep Time: 15 mins **Cook Time:** 0 mins **Total Time:** 15 mins

MAKES 4 SERVINGS

INGREDIENTS

- 1 large apple, diced
- 1 large beet, coarsely grated
- 1 large carrot, coarsely grated
- 1 tbsp chia seeds
- 2 tbsp almonds, chopped
- 2 tbsp lemon juice
- 2 tbsp pumpkin seed oil
- 4 cups mixed greens

INSTRUCTIONS

1. In a medium salad bowl, except for mixed greens, combine all ingredients thoroughly.

2. Into 4 salad plates, divide the mixed greens.
3. Evenly top mixed greens with the salad bowl mixture.

Crab Melt with Avocado and Egg

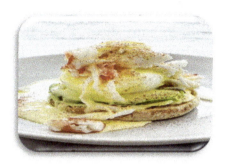

Prep Time: 15 mins **Cook Time:** 15 mins **Total Time:** 30 mins

MAKES 2 SERVINGS

INGREDIENTS

- ✓ 2 English muffins, split
- ✓ 3 tablespoons butter, divided
- ✓ 2 tomatoes, cut into slices
- ✓ 1 (4-ounce) can lump crabmeat
- ✓ 6 ounces sliced or shredded cheddar cheese
- ✓ 4 large eggs
- ✓ Kosher salt
- ✓ 2 large avocados, halved, pitted, and cut into slices
- ✓ Microgreens, for garnish

INSTRUCTIONS

1. Preheat the broiler. Toast the English muffin halves. Place the toasted halves, cut-side up, on a baking sheet.

Spread 1½ teaspoons of butter evenly over each half, allowing the butter to melt into the crevices.
2. Top each with tomato slices, then divide the crab over each, and finish with the cheese. Broil for about 4 minutes until the cheese melts.
3. Meanwhile, in a medium skillet over medium heat, melt the remaining 1 tablespoon of butter, swirling to coat the bottom of the skillet.
4. Crack the eggs into the skillet, giving ample space for each. Sprinkle with salt. Cook for about 3 minutes.
5. Flip the eggs and cook the other side until the yolks are set to your liking. Place 1 egg on each English muffin half. Top with avocado slices and microgreens.

Italian Meatball Soup

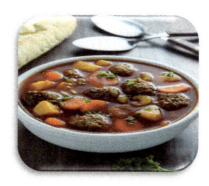

Prep Time: 30 mins **Cook Time:** 30 mins **Total Time:** 1 hr

MAKES 8 SERVINGS

INGREDIENTS

- ✓ 4 cups chicken stock
- ✓ 4 cups water
- ✓ 1 shallot, chopped
- ✓ 2 red bell peppers, cored and diced
- ✓ 1 carrot, diced
- ✓ 1 celery stalk, diced
- ✓ 2 tomatoes, diced
- ✓ 1 cup tomato juice
- ✓ ½ teaspoon dried oregano
- ✓ 1 teaspoon dried basil
- ✓ 1 pound ground chicken
- ✓ 2 tablespoons white rice

- ✓ 1 lemon, juiced
- ✓ Salt and pepper to taste
- ✓ 2 tablespoons chopped parsley

INSTRUCTIONS

1. Combine the stock, water, shallot, bell peppers, carrot, celery, tomatoes, tomato juice, oregano, and basil in a soup pot.
2. Add salt and pepper to taste and cook for 10 minutes.
3. Make the meatballs by mixing the chicken with rice and parsley. Form small meatballs and drop them in the hot soup.
4. Continue cooking for another 15 minutes then add the lemon juice. Serve the soup right away.

Dill Farro

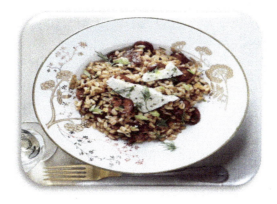

Prep Time: 8 mins **Cook Time:** 40 mins **Total Time:** 48 mins

MAKES 4 SERVINGS

INGREDIENTS

- ✓ 1 cup farro
- ✓ 3 cups beef broth
- ✓ 1 teaspoon salt
- ✓ 1 tablespoon almond butter
- ✓ 1 tablespoon dried dill

INSTRUCTIONS

1. Place the farro in the pan. Add beef broth, dried dill, and salt. Close the lid and bring the mixture to a boil. Then boil it for 35 minutes over medium-low heat.

2. When the time is over, open the lid and add almond butter. Mix up the cooked farro well.

Tuscan Cabbage Soup

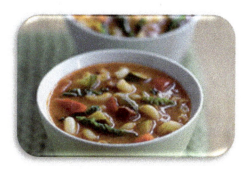

Prep Time: 30 mins **Cook Time:** 30 mins **Total Time:** 1 hr

MAKES 8 SERVINGS

INGREDIENTS

- ✓ 2 tablespoons olive oil
- ✓ 2 sweet onions, chopped
- ✓ 2 carrots, grated
- ✓ 1 celery stalk, chopped
- ✓ 1 can diced tomatoes
- ✓ 1 cabbage, shredded
- ✓ 2 cups vegetable stock
- ✓ 2 cups water
- ✓ 1 lemon, juiced
- ✓ 1 thyme sprig
- ✓ 1 oregano sprig
- ✓ 1 basil sprig
- ✓ Salt and pepper to taste

INSTRUCTIONS

1. Heat the oil in a soup pot and stir in the onions, carrots, and celery. Cook for 5 minutes then stir in the rest of the ingredients.
2. Season with salt and pepper to taste and cook on low heat for 25 minutes.

Creamy Chicken-Spinach Skillet

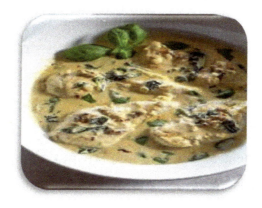

Prep Time: 10 mins **Cook Time:** 17 mins **Total Time:** 27 mins

MAKES 2 SERVINGS

INGREDIENTS

- ✓ Boneless skinless chicken breast, 1 lb.
- ✓ Medium diced onion, 1.
- ✓ Diced roasted red peppers, 12 oz.
- ✓ Chicken stock, 2 ½ cups.
- ✓ Baby spinach leaves, 2 cups.
- ✓ Cooked pasta, 2 cups.
- ✓ Butter, 2 tbsp.
- ✓ Minced garlic cloves, 4. Cream cheese, 7 oz.
- ✓ Salt and pepper, to taste.

INSTRUCTIONS

1. Place a saucepan on medium-high heat for 2 minutes. Add butter and melt for a minute, swirling to coat the pan.
2. Add chicken to a pan, season with pepper and salt to taste. Cook chicken on high heat for 3 minutes per side.
3. Lower heat to medium and stir in onions, red peppers, and garlic. Sauté for 5 minutes and deglaze the pot with a little bit of stock.
4. Whisk in chicken stock and cream cheese. Cook and mix until thoroughly combined.
5. Stir in spinach and adjust seasoning to taste. Cook until spinach is wilted.
6. Serve and enjoy.

Beef and Bulgur Meatballs

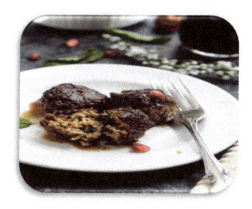

Prep Time: 20 mins **Cook Time:** 28 mins **Total Time:** 48 mins

MAKES 2 SERVINGS

INGREDIENTS

- ✓ ¾ cup uncooked bulgur
- ✓ 1-pound ground beef
- ✓ ¼ cup shallots, minced
- ✓ ¼ cup fresh parsley, minced
- ✓ ½ teaspoon ground allspice
- ✓ ½ teaspoon ground cumin
- ✓ ½ teaspoon ground cinnamon
- ✓ ¼ teaspoon red pepper flakes, crushed
- ✓ Salt, as required
- ✓ 1 tablespoon olive oil

INSTRUCTIONS

1. In a large bowl of cold water, soak the bulgur for about 30 minutes. Drain the bulgur well and then, squeeze with your hands to remove the excess water.
2. In a food processor, add the bulgur, beef, shallot, parsley, spices, salt, and pulse until a smooth mixture is formed.
3. Situate the mixture into a bowl and refrigerate, covered for about 30 minutes. Remove from the refrigerator and make equal-sized balls from the beef mixture.
4. In a large nonstick skillet, heat the oil over medium-high heat and cook the meatballs in 2 batches for about 13-14 minutes, flipping frequently. Serve warm.

Simple and Quick Steak

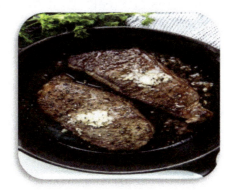

Prep Time: 15 mins **Cook Time:** 10 mins **Total Time:** 25 mins

MAKES 2 SERVINGS

INGREDIENTS

- ✓ ½ lb steak, quality - cut
- ✓ Salt and freshly cracked
- ✓ black pepper

INSTRUCTIONS

1. Switch on the air fryer, set the frying basket in it, then set its temperature to 385°F, and let preheat.
2. Meanwhile, prepare the steaks, and for this, season steaks with salt and freshly cracked black pepper on both sides.
3. When the air fryer has preheated, add prepared steaks to the fryer basket, shut it with a lid and cook for 15

minutes.
4. When done, transfer steaks to a dish and then serve immediately.
5. For meal prepping, evenly divide the steaks between two heatproof containers, close them with a lid and refrigerate for up to 3 days until ready to serve.
6. When ready to eat, reheat steaks into the microwave until hot and then serve.

Mediterranean Grilled Pork Chops

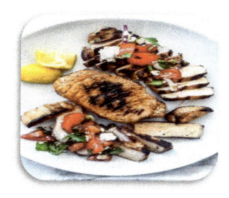

Prep Time: 1 day & 15 mins **Cook Time:** 20 mins **Total Time:** 1 day & 35 mins

MAKES 6 SERVINGS

INGREDIENTS

- ✓ 2 pork chops
- ✓ ¼ cup olive oil
- ✓ 2 yellow onions, sliced
- ✓ 2 garlic cloves, minced
- ✓ 2 teaspoons mustard
- ✓ 1 teaspoon sweet paprika
- ✓ Salt and black pepper, to taste
- ✓ ½ teaspoon oregano, dried
- ✓ ½ teaspoon thyme dried
- ✓ A pinch of cayenne pepper

INSTRUCTIONS

1. In a small bowl, mix oil with garlic, mustard, paprika, black pepper, oregano, thyme, and cayenne, and whisk well.
2. In a bowl, combine onions with meat and mustard mix, toss to coat, cover, and keep in the fridge for 1 day.
3. Place meat on a preheated grill pan over medium-high heat, season with salt, and cook for 10 minutes on each side.
4. Meanwhile, heat a pan over medium heat, add marinated onions, stir and sauté for 4 minutes. Divide pork chops on plates, then add sautéed onions on top and serve.

Four-Cheese Zucchini Noodle with Basil Pesto

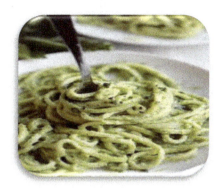

Prep Time: 10 mins **Cook Time:** 15 mins **Total Time:** 25 mins

MAKES 2 SERVINGS

INGREDIENTS

- ✓ 4 cups zucchini noodles
- ✓ 4 oz Mascarpone cheese
- ✓ 1/8 cup Romano cheese
- ✓ 2 tbsp grated parmesan cheese
- ✓ ¼ tsp salt
- ✓ ½ tsp cracked black pepper
- ✓ 2 1/8 tsp ground nutmeg
- ✓ 1/8 cup basil pesto
- ✓ ½ cup shredded mozzarella cheese 1 tbsp olive oil

INSTRUCTIONS

1. Switch on the oven, then set its temperature to 400°F and let it preheat. Meanwhile, place zucchini noodles in a heatproof bowl and microwave at high heat setting for 3 minutes, set aside until required.
2. Take another heatproof bowl, add all cheeses in it, except for mozzarella, season with salt, black pepper, and nutmeg, and microwave at high heat setting for 1 minute until cheese has melted.
3. Whisk the cheese mixture, add cooked zucchini noodles in it along with basil pesto and mozzarella cheese and fold until well mixed.
4. Take a casserole dish, grease it with oil, add zucchini noodles mixture in it, and then bake for 10 minutes until done.
5. Serve straight away.

Pork and Greens Salad

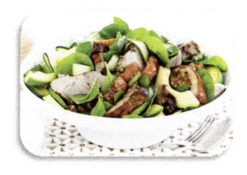

Prep Time: 10 mins **Cook Time:** 15 mins **Total Time:** 25 mins

MAKES 4 SERVINGS

INGREDIENTS

- ✓ 1-pound pork chops, boneless and cut into strips
- ✓ 8 ounces white mushrooms, sliced
- ✓ ½ cup Italian dressing
- ✓ 6 cups mixed salad greens
- ✓ 6 ounces jarred artichoke hearts, drained
- ✓ Salt and black pepper to the taste
- ✓ ½ cup basil, chopped
- ✓ 1 tablespoon olive oil

INSTRUCTIONS

1. Heat a pan with the oil over medium-high heat, add the pork, and brown for 5 minutes. Add the mushrooms, stir

and sauté for 5 minutes more.
2. Add the dressing, artichokes, salad greens, salt, pepper, and basil, cook for 4-5 minutes, divide everything into bowls and serve.

Mustard Chops with Apricot-basil Relish

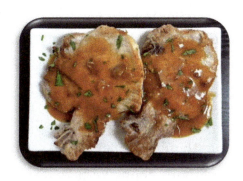

Prep Time: 12 mins **Cook Time:** 12 min **Total Time:** 24 mins

MAKES 4 SERVINGS

INGREDIENTS

- ¼ cup basil, finely shredded
- ¼ cup olive oil
- ½ cup mustard
- ¾ lb. fresh apricots, stone removed, and fruit diced
- 1 shallot, diced small
- 1 tsp ground cardamom
- 3 tbsp raspberry vinegar
- 4 pork chops
- Pepper and salt

INSTRUCTIONS

1. Make sure that pork chops are defrosted well. Season with pepper and salt. Slather both sides of each pork chop with mustard. Preheat grill to medium-high fire.
2. In a medium bowl, mix cardamom, olive oil, vinegar, basil, shallot, and apricots. Toss to combine and season with pepper and salt, mixing once again.
3. Grill chops for 5-6 minutes per side. As you flip, baste with mustard. Serve pork chops with the Apricot-Basil relish and enjoy.

Slow Cooked Mediterranean Pork

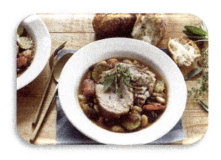

Prep Time: 20 hr **Cook Time:** 8 hr **Total Time:** 28 hr

MAKES 6 SERVINGS

INGREDIENTS

- ✓ 3 pounds pork shoulder - boneless
- ✓ ¼ cup olive oil
- ✓ 2 teaspoons oregano, dried
- ✓ ¼ cup lemon juice
- ✓ 2 teaspoons mustard
- ✓ 2 teaspoons mint, chopped 3 garlic cloves, minced
- ✓ 2 teaspoons pesto sauce
- ✓ Salt and black pepper to taste

INSTRUCTIONS

1. In a bowl, mix olive oil with lemon juice, oregano, mint, mustard, garlic, pesto, salt, and pepper then whisk well.

2. Rub pork with marinade, cover, and keep in a cold place for 10 hours. Flip pork shoulder and then leave aside for 10 more hours.
3. Transfer to your slow cooker along with the marinade juices, cover, and cook on low for 8 hours. Uncover, slice, divide between plates and serve.

Hearty Beef Ragu

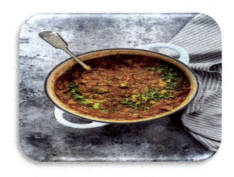

Prep Time: 10 mins **Cook Time:** 50 mins **Total Time:** 60 mins

MAKES 4 SERVINGS

INGREDIENTS

- ✓ 1 1/2 lbs beef steak, diced
- ✓ 1 1/2 cup beef stock
- ✓ 1 tbsp coconut amino
- ✓ 14 oz can tomatoes, chopped
- ✓ 1/2 tsp ground cinnamon
- ✓ 1 tsp dried oregano
- ✓ 1 tsp dried thyme
- ✓ 1 tsp dried basil
- ✓ 1 tsp paprika
- ✓ 1 bay leaf
- ✓ 1 tbsp garlic, chopped
- ✓ 1/2 tsp cayenne pepper
- ✓ 1 celery stick, diced

- ✓ 1 carrot, diced
- ✓ 1 onion, diced
- ✓ 2 tbsp olive oil
- ✓ 1/4 tsp pepper
- ✓ 1 1/2 tsp sea salt

INSTRUCTIONS

1. Add oil into the instant pot, then set the pot on sauté mode. Add celery, carrots, onion, and salt and sauté for 5 minutes. Add meat and remaining ingredients and stir everything well. Seal pot with lid and cook on high for 30 minutes.
2. Allow releasing pressure naturally for 10 minutes then release remaining using quick release. Remove lid.
3. Shred meat using a fork. Set pot on sauté mode and cook for 10 minutes. Stir every 2-3 minutes.
4. Serve and enjoy.

Turkey Meatballs

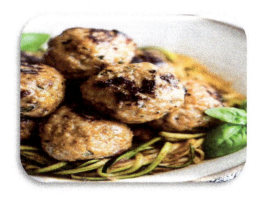

Prep Time: 10 mins **Cook Time:** 25 mins **Total Time:** 35 mins

MAKES 2 SERVINGS

INGREDIENTS

- ✓ Diced yellow onion, ¼
- ✓ Diced artichoke hearts, 14 oz.
- ✓ Ground turkey, 1 lb.
- ✓ Dried parsley, 1 tsp.
- ✓ Oil, 1 tsp.
- ✓ Chopped basil, 4 tbsp.
- ✓ Pepper and salt, to taste.

INSTRUCTIONS

1. Grease the baking sheet and preheat the oven to 3500 F.

2. On medium heat, place a nonstick medium saucepan, sauté artichoke hearts, and diced onions for 5 minutes or until onions are soft.
3. Meanwhile, in a big bowl, mix parsley, basil, and ground turkey with your hands. Season to taste.
4. Once the onion mixture has cooled, add it into the bowl and mix thoroughly.
5. With an ice cream scooper, scoop ground turkey and form balls.
6. Place on a prepared cooking sheet, pop in the oven and bake until cooked around 15-20 minutes.
7. Remove from pan, serve and enjoy

Garlic Caper Beef Roast

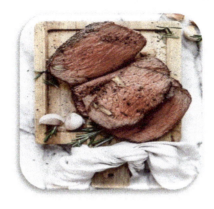

Prep Time: 10 mins **Cook Time:** 40 mins **Total Time:** 50 mins

MAKES 4 SERVINGS

INGREDIENTS

- 2 lbs beef roast, cubed
- 1 tbsp fresh parsley, chopped
- 1 tbsp capers, chopped
- 1 tbsp garlic, minced 1 cup chicken stock
- 1/2 tsp dried rosemary
- 1/2 tsp ground cumin 1 onion, chopped
- 1 tbsp olive oil Pepper

INSTRUCTIONS

1. Add oil into the instant pot and set the pot on sauté mode, then add garlic and onion and sauté for 5 minutes.

2. Add meat and cook until brown.
3. Add remaining ingredients and stir well.
4. Seal pot with lid and cook on high for 30 minutes.
5. Once done, allow to release pressure naturally. Remove lid. Stir well and serve.

Kale Sprouts and Lamb

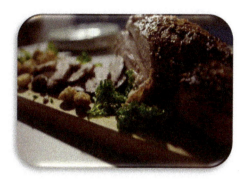

Prep Time: 10 mins **Cook Time:** 30 mins **Total Time:** 40 mins

MAKES 2 SERVINGS

INGREDIENTS

- ✓ 2 lbs. lamb, cut into chunks
- ✓ 1 tbsp. parsley, chopped
- ✓ 2 tbsp. olive oil
- ✓ 1 cup kale, chopped
- ✓ 1 cup Brussels sprouts, halved
- ✓ 1 cup beef stock
- ✓ Pepper Salt

INSTRUCTIONS

1. Add all ingredients into the inner pot of the instant pot and stir well.
2. Seal pot with lid and cook on high for 30 minutes.

3. Once done, allow to release pressure naturally. Remove lid.
4. Serve and enjoy.

Beanless Beef Chili

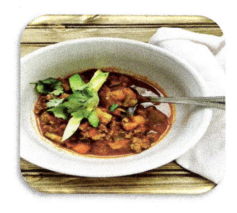

Prep Time: 10 mins **Cook Time:** 20 mins **Total Time:** 30 mins

MAKES 4 SERVINGS

INGREDIENTS

- ✓ 1 lb ground beef
- ✓ 1/2 tsp dried rosemary
- ✓ 1/2 tsp paprika
- ✓ 1 tsp garlic powder
- ✓ 1/2 tsp chili powder
- ✓ 1/2 cup chicken broth
- ✓ 1 cup heavy cream
- ✓ 1 tbsp olive oil
- ✓ 1 tsp garlic, minced
- ✓ 1 small onion, chopped
- ✓ 1 bell pepper, chopped
- ✓ 2 cups tomatoes, diced

- ✓ Pepper
- ✓ Salt

INSTRUCTIONS

1. Add oil into the instant pot and set the pot on sauté mode, then add meat, bell pepper, and onion and sauté for 5 minutes.
2. Add remaining ingredients except for heavy cream and stir well. Seal pot with lid and cook on high for 5 minutes.
3. Once done, release pressure using quick release. Remove lid.
4. Add heavy cream and stir well and cook on sauté mode for 10 minutes. Serve and enjoy.

Classic Chicken Cooking with Tomatoes and Tapenade

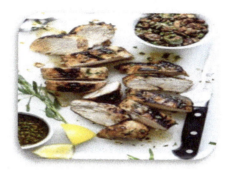

Prep Time: 25 mins **Cook Time:** 25 mins **Total Time:** 50 mins

MAKES 2 SERVINGS

INGREDIENTS

- ✓ 4-5 oz. chicken breasts, boneless and skinless
- ✓ ¼-tsp salt (divided)
- ✓ 3-tbsp fresh basil leaves, chopped (divided)
- ✓ 1-tbsp olive oil
- ✓ 1½-cups cherry tomatoes halved
- ✓ ¼-cup olive tapenade

INSTRUCTIONS

1. Arrange the chicken on a sheet of glassine or waxed paper. Sprinkle half of the salt and a third of the basil evenly over the chicken.

2. Press lightly, and flip over the chicken pieces. Sprinkle the remaining salt and another third of the basil. Cover the seasoned chicken with another sheet of waxed paper.
3. By using a meat mallet or rolling pin, pound the chicken to a half-inch thickness.
4. Heat the olive oil in a 12-inch skillet placed over medium-high heat. Add the pounded chicken breasts.
5. Cook for 6 minutes on each side until the chicken turns golden brown with no traces of pink in the middle. Transfer the browned chicken breasts to a platter, and cover to keep them warm.
6. In the same skillet, add the olive tapenade and tomatoes. Cook for 3 minutes until the tomatoes just begin to be tender.
7. To serve, pour over the tomato-tapenade mixture over the cooked chicken breasts, and top with the remaining basil.

Beef Shawarma

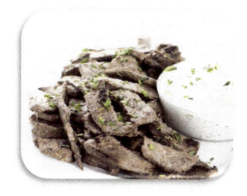

Prep Time: 10 mins **Cook Time:** 10 mins **Total Time:** 20 mins

MAKES 2 SERVINGS

INGREDIENTS

- ✓ 1/2 lb ground beef
- ✓ 1/4 tsp cinnamon
- ✓ 1/2 tsp dried oregano
- ✓ 1 cup cabbage, cut into strips
- ✓ 1/2 cup bell pepper, sliced
- ✓ 1/4 tsp ground coriander
- ✓ 1/4 tsp cumin
- ✓ 1/4 tsp cayenne pepper
- ✓ 1/4 tsp ground allspice
- ✓ 1/2 cup onion, chopped
- ✓ 1/2 tsp salt

INSTRUCTIONS

1. Set instant pot on sauté mode.
2. Add meat to the pot and sauté until brown. Add remaining ingredients and stir well.
3. Seal pot with lid and cook on high for 5 minutes.
4. Once done, release pressure using quick release. Remove lid. Stir and serve.

Mediterranean Lamb Chops

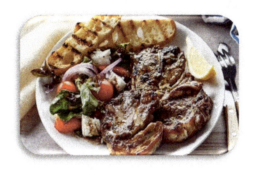

Prep Time: 10 mins **Cook Time:** 10 mins **Total Time:** 20 mins

MAKES 2 SERVINGS

INGREDIENTS

- ✓ 4 lamb shoulder chops, 8 ounces each
- ✓ 2 tablespoons Dijon mustard
- ✓ 2 tablespoons Balsamic vinegar
- ✓ 1 tablespoon garlic, chopped
- ✓ ½ cup olive oil
- ✓ 2 tablespoons shredded fresh basil

INSTRUCTIONS

1. Pat your lamb chop dry using a kitchen towel and arrange them on
2. a shallow glass baking dish.
3. Take a bowl and whisk in Dijon mustard, balsamic vinegar, garlic, pepper, and mix well.

4. Whisk in the oil very slowly into the marinade until the mixture is smooth.
5. Stir in basil.
6. Pour the marinade over the lamb chops and stir to coat both sides well.
7. Cover the chops and allow them to marinate for 1-4 hours (chilled).
8. Take the chops out and leave them for 30 minutes to allow the temperature to reach the normal level.
9. Preheat your grill to medium heat and add oil to the grate.
10. Grill the lamb chops for 5-10 minutes per side until both sides are browned.
11. Once the center of the chop reads 145-degree Fahrenheit, the chops are ready, serve and enjoy!

Lamb and Beet Meatballs

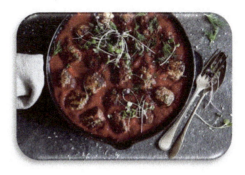

Prep Time: 5 mins **Cook Time:** 20 mins **Total Time:** 25 mins

MAKES 4 SERVINGS

INGREDIENTS

- ✓ 1 tablespoon olive oil
- ✓ 1 (8 oz.) package beets, cooked
- ✓ 6 oz. ground lamb
- ✓ 1/2 cup bulgur, uncooked
- ✓ 1 teaspoon ground cumin
- ✓ 1/2 cup cucumber, grated
- ✓ 1/2 cup sour cream, reduced-fat
- ✓ 2 tablespoons fresh mint, thinly sliced
- ✓ 2 tablespoons fresh lemon juice
- ✓ 1 oz. almond flour
- ✓ 4 cups mixed baby greens
- ✓ 3/4 teaspoon kosher salt
- ✓ 3/4 teaspoon freshly ground black pepper

INSTRUCTIONS

1. Preheat the oven to 425F.
2. Add the beets to a food processor and pulse until finely chopped, Then combine the chopped beets with bulgur, lamb, cumin, ½ teaspoon of salt, pepper, and almond flour in a bowl.
3. Divide the lamb mixture and shape it into 12 meatballs.
4. Heat the oil in a skillet over medium-high heat, then add it into prepared meatballs. Cook until nicely browned on all sides, for about 4 minutes.
5. Transfer the browned meatballs to the preheated oven and bake until well cooked, about 8 minutes.
6. Combine the remaining ¼ teaspoon of salt with cucumber, juice, mint, and sour cream in a bowl, then divide the greens among the serving plates.
7. Top the greens with the meatballs evenly and serve with the cucumber mixture. Enjoy!

Beef and Potatoes

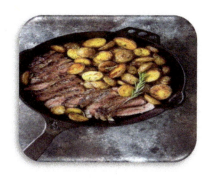

Prep Time: 15 mins **Cook Time:** 20 mins **Total Time:** 35 mins

MAKES 6 BOWLS

INGREDIENTS

- ✓ 1 1/2 lb. stew beef, sliced into cubes
- ✓ 2 teaspoons mixed dried herbs (thyme, sage)
- ✓ 4 potatoes, cubed
- ✓ 10 oz. mushrooms
- ✓ 1 ½ cups red wine

INSTRUCTIONS

1. Set the Instant Pot to sauté. Add 1 tablespoon olive oil and cook the beef until brown on all sides. Add the rest of the ingredients.
2. Season with salt and pepper. Pour in 1 ½ cups water into the pot. Mix well. Cover the pot. Set it to manual. Cook at

high pressure for 20 minutes. Release the pressure naturally.

Beef and Chili Mix

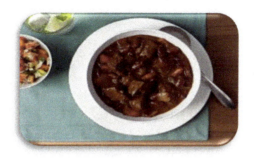

Prep Time: 15 mins **Cook Time:** 16 mins **Total Time:** 31 mins

MAKES 4 SERVINGS

INGREDIENTS

- ✓ 2 green chili peppers
- ✓ 8 oz beef flank steak
- ✓ 1 teaspoon salt
- ✓ 2 tablespoons olive oil
- ✓ 1 teaspoon apple cider vinegar

INSTRUCTIONS

1. Pour olive oil into the skillet. Place the flank steak in the oil and roast it for 3 minutes from each side. Then sprinkle the meat with salt and apple cider vinegar.
2. Chop the chili peppers and add them to the skillet. Fry the beef for 10 minutes more. Stir it from time to time.

Salmon and Eggs

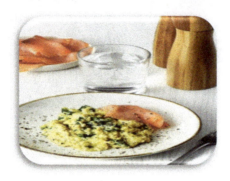

Prep Time: 5 mins **Cook Time:** 10 mins **Total Time:** 15 mins

MAKES 2 SERVINGS

INGREDIENTS

- ✓ 2 eggs
- ✓ 1 lb. salmon, seasoned and cooked
- ✓ 1 cup celery, chopped
- ✓ 1 onion, chopped
- ✓ 1 tablespoon olive oil
- ✓ Salt and pepper to taste

INSTRUCTIONS

1. Whisk the eggs in a bowl. Add celery, onion, salt, and pepper. Add the oil to a round baking tray and pour in the egg mixture.

2. Place in air fryer on 300°Fahrenheit. Let it cook for 10-minutes. When done, serve with cooked salmon.

Grilled Calamari with Lemon Juice

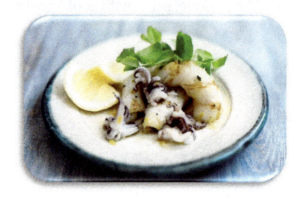

Prep Time: 10 mins **Cook Time:** 15 mins **Total Time:** 25 mins

MAKES 2 SERVINGS

INGREDIENTS

- ¼ c. dried cranberries
- ¼ c. extra virgin olive oil
- ¼ c. olive oil
- ¼ c. sliced almonds 1/3 c. fresh lemon juice
- ¾ c. blueberries
- 1 ½ lbs. or 700 g. cleaned calamari tube
- 1 granny smith apple, sliced thinly
- 2 tbsps. apple cider vinegar
- 6 c. fresh spinach
- Grated pepper
- Sea salt

INSTRUCTIONS

1. In a medium bowl, mix lemon juice, apple cider vinegar, and extra virgin olive oil to make a sauce. Season with pepper and salt to taste, then mix well.
2. Turn on the grill to medium fire and let the grates heat up for 1-2 minutes.
3. In a separate bowl, add olive oil and the calamari tube. Season calamari generously with pepper and salt.
4. Place calamari onto heated grate and grill for 2-3 minutes on each side or until opaque.
5. Meanwhile, combine almonds, cranberries, blueberries, spinach, and the thinly sliced apple in a large salad bowl. Toss to mix.
6. Remove cooked calamari from grill and transfer on a chopping board. Cut into ¼-inch thick rings and throw into the salad bowl.
7. Sprinkle with already prepared sauce. Toss well to coat and serve.

Tasty Tuna with Roast Potatoes

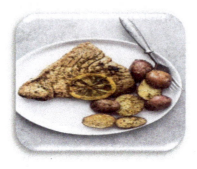

Prep Time: 5 mins **Cook Time:** 30 mins **Total Time:** 35 mins

MAKES 4 SERVINGS

INGREDIENTS

- ✓ 4 medium potatoes
- ✓ 1 teaspoon olive oil
- ✓ ½ tablespoon capers
- ✓ Salt and pepper to taste
- ✓ 1 green onion, sliced
- ✓ 1 tablespoon Greek yogurt
- ✓ ½ teaspoon chili powder
- ✓ ½ can of tuna in oil, drained
- ✓ 2 boiled eggs, sliced

INSTRUCTIONS

1. Soak the potatoes in water for 30-minutes. Pat dry with kitchen towel. Brush the potatoes with olive oil. Place

potatoes in air fryer and air fry for 30- minutes at 355°Fahrenheit. Put tuna in a bowl with yogurt and chili powder, mix well. Add half of the green onion plus salt and pepper. Slit potatoes length-wise. Stuff tuna mixture in middle of potatoes and place on a serving plate. Sprinkle with chili powder and remaining green onions over potatoes.
2. Serve with capers and a salad of your choice and topped with boiled egg slices.

Seafood Risotto

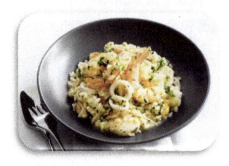

Prep Time: 15 mins **Cook Time:** 30 mins **Total Time:** 45 mins

MAKES 4 SERVINGS

INGREDIENTS

- ✓ 6 cups vegetable broth
- ✓ 3 tablespoons extra-virgin olive oil
- ✓ 1 large onion, chopped
- ✓ 3 cloves garlic, minced
- ✓ ½ teaspoon saffron threads
- ✓ 1½ cups arborio rice
- ✓ 1½ teaspoons salt
- ✓ 8 ounces (227 g) shrimp (21 to 25), peeled and deveined
- ✓ 8 ounces (227 g) scallops

INSTRUCTIONS

1. In a large saucepan over medium heat, bring the broth to a

low simmer. In a large skillet over medium heat, cook the olive oil, onion, garlic, and saffron for 3 minutes.
2. Add the rice, salt, and 1 cup of the broth to the skillet. Stir the ingredients together and cook over low heat until most of the liquid is absorbed.
3. Repeat steps with broth, adding ½ cup of broth at a time, and cook until all but ½ cup of the broth is absorbed.
4. Add the shrimp and scallops when you stir in the final ½ cup of broth. Cover and let cook for 10 minutes. Serve warm.

Coconut Shrimp

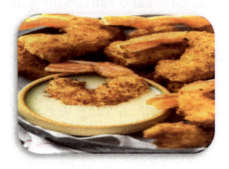

Prep Time: 5 mins **Cook Time:** 10 mins **Total Time:** 15 mins

MAKES 4 SERVINGS

INGREDIENTS

- ✓ 1 cup breadcrumbs
- ✓ 1 cup dried coconut, unsweetened
- ✓ 1 cup almond flour
- ✓ Sea salt to taste
- ✓ 2 lbs. shrimp
- ✓ 1 cup egg whites

INSTRUCTIONS

1. In a mixing bowl, combine coconut and breadcrumbs. Season lightly with sea salt. In another bowl, add flour, and in a third bowl, add egg whites. Preheat your air fryer to 340°Fahrenheit. Dip each shrimp into the flour, egg whites, then the breadcrumbs.

2. Cook the shrimps for 10-minutes and serve with preferred dipping sauce.

Almond-Crusted Swordfish

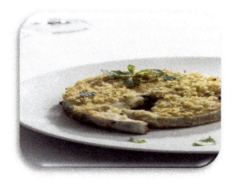

Prep Time: 15 mins **Cook Time:** 15 mins **Total Time:** 30 mins

MAKES 4 SERVINGS

INGREDIENTS

- ✓ ½ cup almond flour
- ✓ ¼ cup crushed Marcona almonds
- ✓ ½ to 1 teaspoon salt, divided
- ✓ 2 pounds (907 g) Swordfish, preferably 1 inch thick
- ✓ 1 large egg, beaten (optional)
- ✓ ¼ cup pure apple cider
- ✓ ¼ cup extra-virgin olive oil, plus more for frying
- ✓ 3 to 4 sprigs flat-leaf parsley, chopped
- ✓ 1 lemon, juiced
- ✓ 1 tablespoon Spanish paprika
- ✓ 5 medium baby portobello mushrooms, chopped (optional)

- ✓ 4 or 5 chopped scallions, both green and white parts
- ✓ 3 to 4 garlic cloves, peeled
- ✓ ¼ cup chopped pitted Kalamata olives

INSTRUCTIONS

1. On a dinner plate, spread the flour and crushed Marcona almonds and mix in the salt. Alternately, pour the flour, almonds, and ¼ teaspoon of salt into a large plastic food storage bag.
2. Add the fish and coat it with the flour mixture. If a thicker coat is desired, repeat this step after dipping the fish in the egg (if using).
3. In a measuring cup, combine the apple cider, ¼ cup of olive oil, parsley, lemon juice, paprika, and ¼ teaspoon of salt. Mix well and set aside.
4. In a large, heavy-bottom sauté pan or skillet, pour the olive oil to a depth of ⅛ inch and heat on medium heat.
5. Once the oil is hot, add the fish and brown for 3 to 5 minutes, then turn the fish over and add the mushrooms (If using), scallions, garlic, and olives.
6. Cook for an additional 3 minutes. Once the other side of the fish is brown, remove the fish from the pan and set it aside.
7. Pour the cider mixture into the skillet and mix well with the vegetables. Put the fried fish into the skillet on top of

the mixture and cook with sauce on medium-low heat for 10 minutes, until the fish flakes easily with a fork.
8. Carefully remove the fish from the pan and plate. Spoon the sauce over the fish. Serve with white rice or home-fried potatoes.

Creamy Air Fryer Salmon

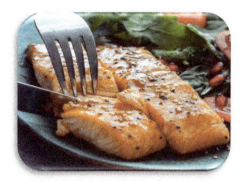

Prep Time: 5 mins **Cook Time:** 10 mins **Total Time:** 15 mins

MAKES 2 SERVINGS

INGREDIENTS

- ✓ ¾ lb. salmon, cut into 6 pieces
- ✓ Salt to taste
- ✓ ¼ cup plain yogurt
- ✓ 1 tablespoon dill, chopped
- ✓ 3 tablespoons light sour cream
- ✓ 1 tablespoon olive oil

INSTRUCTIONS

1. Season the salmon with salt and place it in the air fryer. Drizzle the salmon with olive oil. Air-fry salmon at 285°Fahrenheit and cook for 10-minutes.
2. Mix the dill, yogurt, sour cream, and some salt.

3. Place salmon on the serving dish and drizzle with creamy sauce.

Peanut Butter and Chocolate Balls

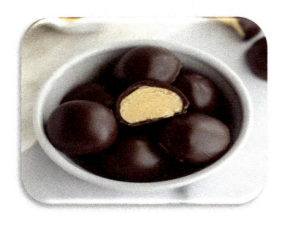

Prep Time: 45 mins **Cook Time:** 0 mins **Total Time:** 45 mins

MAKES 15 BALLS

INGREDIENTS

- ¾ cup creamy peanut butter
- ¼ cup unsweetened cocoa powder
- 2 tablespoons softened almond butter
- ½ teaspoon vanilla extract
- 1¾ cups maple sugar

INSTRUCTIONS

1. Line a baking sheet with parchment paper. Combine all the ingredients in a bowl. Stir to mix well.

2. Divide the mixture into 15 parts and shape each part into a 1-inch ball. Arrange the balls on the baking sheet and refrigerate for at least 30 minutes, then serve chilled.

Peach Cake

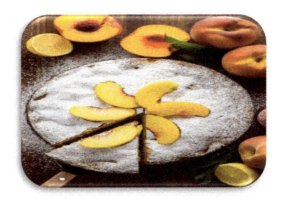

Prep Time: 10 mins **Cook Time:** 35 mins **Total Time:** 45 mins

MAKES 6 SERVINGS

INGREDIENTS

- ½ lb. peaches, pitted and mashed
- ½ teaspoon baking powder
- 1 ¼ cups almond flour
- ½ teaspoon orange extract
- ¼ teaspoon nutmeg, freshly grated
- 2 eggs
- 2 tablespoons Truvia for baking
- 1/3 cup ghee
- ¼ teaspoon ground cinnamon
- 1 teaspoon pure vanilla extract

INSTRUCTIONS

1. Preheat your air-fryer to 310°Fahrenheit. Spritz the cake pan with olive oil cooking spray. In a mixing bowl, beat the ghee with Truvia until creamy. Fold in the egg, mashed peaches, and honey. Then, make the cake batter by mixing the remaining ingredients; now, stir in the peach mixture with the rest of the ingredients.
2. Pour the batter into the cake pan and level the surface of the batter.
3. Bake 35-minutes and enjoy!

Mascarpone and Fig Crostini

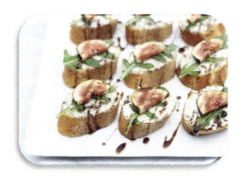

Prep Time: 10 mins **Cook Time:** 10 mins **Total Time:** 20 mins

MAKES 6-8 SERVINGS

INGREDIENTS

- ✓ 1 long French baguette
- ✓ 4 tablespoons (½ stick) salted butter, melted 1
- ✓ (8-ounce) tub mascarpone cheese
- ✓ 1 (12-ounce) jar fig jam or preserves

INSTRUCTIONS

1. Preheat the oven to 350°F. Slice the bread into ¼-inch-thick slices. Layout the sliced bread on a single baking sheet and brush each slice with the melted butter.
2. Put the single baking sheet in the oven and toast the bread for 5 to 7 minutes, just until golden brown.

3. Let the bread cool slightly. Spread about a teaspoon or so of the mascarpone cheese on each piece of bread. Top with a teaspoon or so of the jam. Serve immediately.

Chocolate Mini Cheesecakes

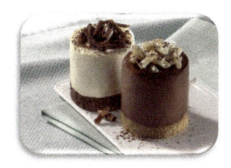

Prep Time: 10 mins **Cook Time:** 18 mins **Total Time:** 28 mins

MAKES 8 SERVINGS

INGREDIENTS

For the crust:

- ✓ 1/3 teaspoon nutmeg, grated
- ✓ 1 tablespoon Truvia
- ✓ ½ cup graham cracker crumbs
- ✓ 1 ½ tablespoon melted butter
- ✓ 1 teaspoon ground cinnamon
- ✓ A pinch of salt

For the Cheesecake:

- ✓ 2 eggs
- ✓ 1 ½ cups chocolate chips
- ✓ 1 ½ tablespoon sour cream

- ✓ 1 package soft cheese
- ✓ 2 tablespoons Truvia for baking
- ✓ ½ teaspoon vanilla essence

INSTRUCTIONS

1. Firstly, line eight cups of the mini muffin pan with paper liners. To make the crust, mix the graham cracker crumbs with 1 tablespoon Truvia, cinnamon, nutmeg, and salt. Now, add the melted butter to moisten the crumb mixture. Divide the crumb mixture among the muffin cups and press gently to make even layers.
2. In another bowl, whip the soft cheese, sour cream, and 2 tablespoons Truvia until smooth. Fold the eggs and vanilla essence into the mix. Divide half of the chocolate chips among the prepared muffin cups. Then, add the cheese mix to each muffin cup. Place another layer using remaining chocolate chips. Bake for 18-minutes at 345°Fahrenheit. Bake in batches, if needed.
3. To finish, transfer mini cheesecakes to a cooling rake.

CPSIA information can be obtained
at www.ICGtesting.com
Printed in the USA
BVHW050239120321
602276BV00012B/1215